SLEEPING DISORDER:

SYMPTOMS, CAUSES

AND NATURAL

REMEDIES

OVERVIEW

For many children, men and women, getting a good night's sleep is a difficult feat - an anxiety related sleep disorder can make it difficult to fall asleep, and stay asleep. While a warm bath and a glass of milk might seem like the simple solution, those who suffer from recurring symptoms associated with anxiety know that it can take a lot more than a hot bath to cure this ailment. While lots of people report having the occasional bad nights sleep, for many people who experience long-term sleep disorders and anxiety, it is a chronic problem.

Anxiety Disorders & Sleep The term "anxiety disorder" encompasses a group of illnesses that include obsessive-compulsive disorder, panic disorder, post-traumatic stress disorder, social anxiety disorder, general anxiety disorder and phobias. These are all medical conditions, which can be treated. These disorders can result from stress and anxiety, and can present themselves in a variety of ways. Some people might experience insomnia, which is the clinical term for when someone is unable to fall asleep or stay sleep. This could include waking up too early in the morning, or waking up feeling un-refreshed and drowsy. There are many common sleep disorders, such as sleep walking, sleep apnea and narcolepsy (falling asleep spontaneously). So, what do sleep disorders have to do with anxiety disorders? Research has shown that anxiety can cause a this disorder - but, interestingly, a sleep disorder can also cause anxiety. What came first? In many cases, it is a vicious cycle. Some antidepressants and anxiety medications can cause sleeping problems; while a lack of sleep has been proven to cause anxiety, depression, and psychiatric disorders. It is always advisable to exert caution when trying new medications, especially sleep inducing pills, which can be addictive. Treatment for Anxiety and Sleep Disorders Stress reduction is a major factor in the treatment of anxiety sleep disorders. Regular exercise can decrease stress, and the practice of yoga and meditation can help individuals to relax. If you are having a sleeping disorder, speak to your doctor. He or she may recommend that you visit a sleep disorder clinic, where they specialize in sleep problems. Typically, the treatment for will include relaxation techniques, medication, and cognitive-behavior therapy. What Can I Do? There are many things that can be done at home to reduce overall levels of stress and anxiety. These stress-reducers include exercise and yoga, prioritizing seven to nine hours per night for sleep, and establishing a regular bedtime routine. Avoiding stimulants like caffeine, chocolate, and nicotine before sleep can help with sleeping disorders. It is also recommended to avoid doing other activities in bed, such as work or watching TV. Anxiety can certainly result in sleep disorders, and it is important to recognize when there is a problem so that one can begin treatment as early as possible. Speak to your doctor about the sorts of treatments that are available to you to help you live a better life, with an anxiety-related sleep disorder.

What Are Sleep Disorders?

Sleep disorders are conditions that impair your sleep or prevent you from getting restful sleep and, as a result, can cause daytime sleepiness and other symptoms. Everyone can experience problems with sleep from time to time. However, you might have a sleep disorder if:

• You regularly experience difficulty sleeping.

• You are often tired during the day even though you slept for at least seven hours the night before.

- You have a reduced or impaired ability to perform regular daytime activities.

There are more than 100 million Americans of all ages who are not getting an adequate amount of sleep. Sleep is very important. Not getting enough sleep can have untoward consequences on school and work performance, interpersonal relationships, health and safety.

How Much Sleep Is Necessary?

Experts generally recommend that adults sleep at least seven to nine hours per night, although some people require more and others require less.

A recent National Sleep Foundation Sleep in America poll found that adults (ages 18-54) sleep an average of 6.4 hours per night on weekdays and 7.7 hours on weekends. The poll showed a downward trend in sleep time over the past several years. People sleeping less hours tend to use the internet at night or bring work home from the office.

The National Sleep Foundation also reported that older adults (age 55-84) average seven hours of sleep on weekdays and 7.1 hours on weekends. Sleep is most often disturbed by the need to use the bathroom and physical pain or discomfort in older adults.

A downward trend in sleep time has also been observed in children. Optimal sleep time varies by age. An earlier Sleep in America poll found a discrepancy between recommended and actual sleep time in children, with actual sleep time 1.5 to two hours less than recommended. Caffeine consumption caused a loss of three to five hours of sleep and having a television in the bedroom contributed to a loss of two hours of sleep each week in children.

What happens when a person doesn't get enough sleep?

Not getting the proper amount or quality of sleep leads to more than just feeling tired. Sleepiness interferes with cognitive function, which can lead to learning disabilities in children, memory impairment in people of all ages, personality changes and depression.

People who are deprived of sleep experience difficulty making decisions, irritability, have problems with performance, and slower reaction times, placing them at risk for automobile and work-related accidents. Sleep loss can also adversely affect life by contributing to the development of obesity, diabetes and heart disease.

Who Is More Likely To Have A Sleep Disorder?

Disorders associated with daytime sleepiness affect females more than males.

Sleep Disorders in Children

Many children experience sleep disorders. They vary from night terrors and sleep walking to serious breathing disorders. The most common causes of daytime sleep are insufficient sleep at night and abnormal or other unhygienic sleep practices. About 30% of children have sleep disorders in their childhood. The sleep-environment history of a person is a very important factor when diagnosing sleep disorders. A child cycles between light and deep sleep phases during sleep. During each light sleep, there is more chance for the child to wake up. Normally, school aged children need 9 to 12 hours of sleep at night. If a child can go to bed, fall asleep, wake up easily and not felt tired during the day, then he is getting enough sleep. The symptoms of children's sleep disorders are often different than the symptoms of an adult. So it is important that for parents and caregivers give special attention when treating a child's sleep disorders. The common symptoms include falling asleep in the classroom, during conversations, during a journey, or while watching the television or reading a book. Carelessness and mood swings are often symptoms of sleep disorders. The most common sleep disorders include nightmares/night terrors, sleepwalking/talking, bruxism, head banging or rolling and bedwetting (enuresis.) A child's fear of the dark can worsen sleep disorders. This often results in nightmares. Sleepwalking, also called somnambulism) is a harmless disorder if the parents can make the environment safe. Talking while asleep is also harmless. Bruxism (grinding and gnashing the teeth during sleep) is an annoying sleep disturber. It can even lead to dental problems. Most children are head rollers or head bangers during their sleep. It is another harmless disorder that would normally disappear before adolescence. It is advisable to consult a doctor in case of prolonged occurrence of bedwetting. The most common breathing disorder derived from sleep disorders is apnea (OSA). It is very common in preschool-age children. Its symptoms are snoring, restless sleep, breathing interruption, chronic mouth breathing, difficulty awakening, bedwetting and problems with school performance. Pediatric sleep disorders are mostly treatable diseases.

Sleep And Men

For many men, sleep is just one more thing at the bottom of the list of all that needs to be done in a day. It seems like wasted time that prevents them from getting any work done. These wrong ideas about sleep keep men from tapping into the power of a well-rested mind and body.

In reality, sleeping is your most valuable activity of the day. The more you invest in your sleep, the bigger return you will see in everything else that you do. Sleep is not wasted time spent doing nothing. It is a time when your body is actively recharging itself and preparing for the next day. Sleeping well enables you to feel, think, and perform better. It allows you to maximize your time and your energy during the day. The best way to do all that you want to do is to make sure that you get the sleep your body needs.

What Keeps Men From Getting Enough Sleep?

I.   Lack of Awareness

Many men simply don't realize that they need more sleep. They view sleepiness as a positive sign that they must be working hard. They get used to being tired, and they think that's the way it's supposed to be. They believe that they just have to fight through it.

Every person has their own need for sleep. This need varies from one person to another. On average, most adults need seven to eight hours of sleep each night to feel alert and well rested. Many men do not get this much sleep on a regular basis. As a result, they are not able to function at a maximum level of energy and concentration.

The following are signs that you are not getting enough sleep:

• You feel tired and lack energy during the day.

• You have a hard time paying attention during meetings.

- You are unmotivated and have trouble "getting going."

- You are irritable, grouchy or lose your temper easily.

- You must use an alarm clock to wake up on time in the morning.

- You start to doze off when you are driving a car.

Sleeping in later is not an option for most people who have to be at work early in the morning. Not too many employers are going to let you take a daytime nap, either. The solution is to go to bed earlier. Plan to go to bed early enough so that you will have seven to eight hours before you have to get up in the morning. Set it as a goal and make it a priority. After doing this for a while, you will have a better idea if you need even more than eight hours of sleep, or maybe less than seven, to feel refreshed when you wake up.

Work Demands

A man's job can demand so much of his time that it doesn't leave much room for sleep. In order to get ahead, you may feel like you have to put in extra hours at night, go in on the weekends, or be the first one there in the morning. A long commute through heavy traffic may take away even more of your free time. Even when you are away from the job, your work can consume your time. You may have paperwork that you have to finish at home. Your cell phone won't stop ringing. Your e-mail needs to be constantly checked. Before you are even aware of it, time has flown by and it is well past your normal bedtime.

The stress and pressure of a job can also affect your sleep. Each night might be filled with worries and anxiety about what is going to happen tomorrow. Your body wants to rest, but your mind won't stop spinning. As a result, you toss and turn in bed late into the night. Maybe you fall asleep quickly but wake up in the middle of the night and can't go back to sleep. Before long, the alarm clock says that it's time to get up and start the day.

You need to try your best to leave your work at work. As much as it is possible, don't bring your job home with you. You need time away to relax both your body and your mind. Set boundaries and protect your personal free time. This will be very hard if you work from home. You will need to find ways to get out of the house to relax and unwind. You should also find a way to get your worries out of your system during the day. Talk to one of your buddies about them. Release them at the gym. Simply make sure that your bed is a place of rest, not worry.

Full Schedules

Many men have schedules that are filled with much more than just work. They go to the gym for a regular workout. They play sports or go see the local teams in action. They work on the car or on projects around the house. They are involved with a civic group, fraternal order, or local church. Single men go on dates or out on the town with friends. Married men pick up the kids from practice or help them with their homework. The list of people, places, and things that can exhaust a man's time is endless.

The key is to set priorities and balance your time. Take an honest look at your schedule to see if you are doing too much. Some things are more urgent than others. Not everything has to be done today, and not everything has to be done by you. Some things that are important can still be re-arranged so that you make better use of your time. Other things may need to be scaled back so you don't do them as often or for so long. Still other things that are not a high priority may need to be eliminated right now. You can always come back to them if you free up more time in your schedule down the road. As you are deciding which activities are important, make sure that sleeping is one of them. Put it at the top of your list, not at the bottom.

Life Changes

Life is full of changes that can have a big impact upon how you sleep. Some changes you expect, but others catch you by surprise. Negative changes will tend to disturb your sleep the most. But positive changes can affect you too. Along with excitement, good changes bring new duties and stress that can keep you up at night.

Examples of these kinds of changes include the following:

- Getting married

- Having a baby

- Starting a new job

- Moving

Examples of the negative changes that can greatly affect your sleep include the following:

- Losing a loved one

- Losing a job

- Getting divorced

- Being in an auto accident

- Having a major illness

- Having a lawsuit filed against you

- Making a bad investment

These changes can cause you to have feelings of depression. For many men, it begins so slowly that they never become aware that they are depressed. Over time, it can progress to the point where despair is just a normal part of their lives.

Depression can greatly disrupt the quality of your sleep. You might lie in bed tossing and turning late into the night. You also might sleep for a long time with no motivation to get out of bed. As poor sleep progresses, men stop taking care of their bodies in other ways. They stop eating and exercising regularly. They abuse alcohol and drugs. Overall, they may lose their usual interest and pleasure in the normal activities of daily life.

Men are more likely to keep these feelings of depression trapped inside. They don't often deal with them openly. In some cases, these feelings one day explode in a violent outburst. Depressed men often turn this violence on themselves. Statistics show that men are four times as likely as women to kill themselves.

Many men resist seeking help from a counselor. They fear that people will think something is "wrong" with them. They need to understand that these feelings are perfectly normal. But while they are normal, they can also be hazardous to their health. If you are struggling with feelings of depression, then at least start by talking to a spouse, friend, doctor or minister. Any of them can help you decide if you need to see a counselor. Don't fight this battle alone.

Bad Habits

Men can develop a number of habits that cause bad sleep. The use of alcohol, nicotine, and caffeine can all affect your sleep. You should avoid these substances in the afternoon and at night. Consuming them too close to your bedtime can keep you from sleeping well.

You may also eat big meals or exercise just before you go to bed. Both of these habits can also disturb your sleep. This can be hard to avoid if you have a lot going on in the evenings. If needed, you might want to eat a bigger meal at lunch and a smaller meal for dinner. To fit in your workout, perhaps you can try to exercise before work or on your lunch break.

Men also may keep an irregular sleep schedule. They go to bed and wake up at different times every day. This can disrupt your internal body clock and keep you from sleeping soundly. You should try to wake up at the same time every day. This includes weekends and holidays. This will help to keep your internal clock set at the right time. Try to avoid sleeping in later on the weekends to catch up on lost sleep. Instead, go to bed earlier at night when you are tired. You should also keep naps to less than one hour. Be sure to take them in the early afternoon so you are not wide awake at bedtime.

Medical Conditions

Many medical conditions can keep you from being able to sleep well. Some of these are only temporary. A sprained ankle, the flu, or minor surgery will disrupt your sleep for a short while. Other problems may stay with you for the rest of your life. These illnesses and medical conditions become more common as you grow older.

The following are examples of medical conditions that can greatly disturb your sleep:

- Epilepsy

- Asthma and other respiratory diseases

- Heart disease

- Arthritis

Medications used to treat these and other problems can also hinder you from getting quality sleep. Some drugs might make you jittery and keep you up at night. Others will cause you to be very sleepy during the day. Discuss these medications with your doctor. Changing the dose or when you take the drug might make a big difference for you.

II. What Sleep Disorders Affect Men?

There are many men who are unable to get quality sleep even though they spend enough time in bed each night.

It may take them a long time to fall asleep. Their sleep may be disrupted and broken. They may sleep through the night but still feel tired the next day.

These are all signs of sleep disorders that are common to men. Most men who have a sleep disorder are unaware of it. Even when they are aware, many times they will not seek help for it. Detecting and treating a sleep disorder can cause a dramatic improvement in your sleep. This will allow you to sleep your best at night and feel your best during the day.

The most common sleep disorders that affect men include the following:

Obstructive Sleep Apnea (OSA)

Obstructive sleep apnea (OSA) occurs when the tissue in the back of the throat collapses during sleep. This keeps air from getting in to the lungs. This is very common, because the muscles inside the throat relax as you sleep. Gravity then causes the tongue to fall back and block the airway. It can happen a few times a night or several hundred times per night.

These pauses in breathing briefly wake you up and disturb your sleep. This can cause you to be very tired the next day. Men are twice as likely as women to have OSA. Being overweight and having a large neck size also greatly increase your risk of suffering from it. These men have more fatty tissue in their throat that can block their airway.

The primary signs of OSA are daytime sleepiness and loud snoring. Snoring is due to a partial blockage of the airway during sleep. It tends to increase as you age. There is a range of snoring from simple to severe. Simple, primary snoring is "normal" and is mostly harmless. But loud, severe snoring with gasps and snorts is a cause for concern. Many men do not even know that they snore. It is often a spouse or bed partner who detects the loud snoring problem.

Some men consider snoring to be a badge of honor. It is a sign of true masculinity. But they don't realize that there are dangers that can come along with it. Sleep apnea may make it hard for you to think or concentrate during the day. If left untreated, it may also put you at risk of heart or lung disease, high blood pressure or diabetes.

Talk to your doctor if you snore loudly and are often tired during the day. He may refer you to a sleep specialist to find out if you have sleep apnea. Losing weight and sleeping on one's side may help in some mild cases of OSA. Severe sleep apnea requires medical treatment.

Positive airway pressure (PAP) is the most common way to treat OSA in adults. PAP provides a gentle and steady flow of air through a mask that is worn over the nose. This keeps the airway open and prevents pauses in breathing as you sleep. Surgery or the use of an oral appliance (similar to a sports mouth guard) may be a better option for some people.

Narcolepsy

Narcolepsy is the term used to describe people who suffer from extreme sleepiness. It can cause you to suddenly fall asleep. These "sleep attacks" can happen while eating, walking or driving. Narcolepsy usually starts between the ages of 12 and 20 and can last for your entire life. It does not get better without treatment.

Talk to your doctor if you are so tired that you might fall asleep at any time. He might refer you to a sleep specialist to find out if you have narcolepsy. Medications can be used to treat narcolepsy and help you have a more normal pattern of being asleep and awake.

Delayed Sleep Phase Disorder (DSP)

Busy work and social schedules can cause some men to get in the habit of going to bed very late. Delayed sleep phase disorder (DSP) is when you can only fall asleep a couple hours or more later than normal. This also causes you to have a hard time waking up early in the morning.

Your internal body clock makes you feel sleepy or alert at regular times every day. Everyone's body has this natural timing system. A consistent habit of staying up and sleeping late can throw off the timing of your body clock. This can prevent you from being able to fall asleep at a decent time.

To correct DSP, try to avoid bright light in the late afternoon and evening. Keep the lights in the house dim and make your bedroom dark when you go to sleep. Then get plenty of bright sunlight in the morning and early afternoon. This will help to keep your body clock set at the right time. The key is for your eyes to see the light. They send the signals to your brain that will be used to set your body clock. Your skin does not need to be exposed to the sunlight.

Jet Lag Disorder And Shift Work Disorder

Your work conditions can also cause you to have jet lag or shift work disorders. Men who often travel long distances by airplane suffer from jet lag. A long trip quickly puts you in a place where you need to sleep and wake at a time that is different than what your internal body clock expects. Your body clock does not have time to adjust right away to a new location due to the speed of the travel. This makes it very hard for you to sleep well.

Men who work rotating, early-morning or night shifts often suffer from shift work. Your schedule requires you to work when your body wants to sleep. Then you have to try to sleep when your body expects to be awake. This causes you to have trouble sleeping and to be severely tired.

The use of melatonin supplements has been shown to help some people who suffer from jet lag. Melatonin is a hormone that is released by the brain at night. It seems to play a role in making you sleepy.

Light therapy may also help someone with jet lag or shift work. Light therapy is used to expose your eyes to intense amounts of light. This occurs for a specific and regular length of time. This light is meant to affect your body clock in the same way that sunlight does. Talk to your doctor to see if either melatonin or light therapy might help you sleep better.

Inadequate Sleep Hygiene

This insomnia might also be called "bad sleep habits." It involves the things that you normally do every day. These habits keep your sleep from being refreshing. They can also keep you from feeling alert during the day. These activities are all things that you should be able to control. They include such things as drinking alcohol or caffeine at night, taking long naps during the day, or keeping an irregular sleep schedule. A sleep specialist can use behavioral therapy or sleep hygiene training to help you overcome these bad habits.

III. How Can Men Sleep Better?

Most men will sleep much better if they simply develop the habits of good sleep hygiene. Sleep hygiene consists of basic tips that help you develop a pattern of healthy sleep. See the Resources section of this site to find out how anyone can start down the path to better sleep.

Some men think that drinking alcohol will help them sleep better. Alcohol makes you sleepy and might help you fall asleep faster. But it is also likely to cause you to wake up during the night. Many people wake up too early after drinking alcohol in the evening. This may be a "rebound" from the use of alcohol. It stays in your system for a long time after you have a drink. To improve your sleep, you should not have any alcohol within six hours of your bedtime. You should also limit how much and how often you drink. The heavy use of alcohol can be harmful to your overall health.

Men sometimes see sleeping pills as the answer to their sleep problems.

These drugs can be useful in helping some people sleep better. But pills should not be seen as a long-term solution for better sleep. Doctors rarely prescribe them for more than a few weeks at a time.

You can also find many sleep aids on the shelves of your local drugstore. Most of these use antihistamine, the same ingredient found in many cold medicines. While they can have a positive effect on your sleep, they can also make you very groggy during the day. They should be used with caution.

You should not depend upon drugs to help you sleep on a regular basis. Talk to your doctor about other options that will help improve your sleep.

If you have trouble sleeping for more than a month, talk to your doctor about it. Don't think that it will just go away over time. He may encourage you to visit a sleep specialist to find the source of your sleeping difficulty. Before going to see him, complete a daily sleep diary for two weeks. The sleep diary will help the doctor see your sleeping patterns. This information gives the doctor clues about what is hindering your sleep and how to help you.

Your sleep is too important for you to ignore the signs of trouble. You have too much to gain by seeking help from a doctor. Don't put it off. Your sleep will affect the quality of every other area of your life

Sleep Disorders in Women

How do Sleep Disorders in Women Work?

Women are twice as likely as men to have difficulties falling asleep or staying asleep. Younger women have more sound sleep with fewer disturbances. Some women are prone to sleep problems throughout their reproductive years. Only recently has the medical community focused on women's sleep disorders.

A number of factors may affect women's sleep. Changes in hormonal levels, stress, illness, lifestyle, and sleep environment may impact sleep. Pregnancy- and menstrual-related hormonal fluctuations may affect sleep patterns, mood, and reaction to stress. Many women have premenstrual sleep disturbances. Difficulty falling asleep, nighttime waking, difficulty waking up, and daytime sleepiness all are linked to premenstrual changes. Insomnia (sleeplessness) is one of the most common symptoms of premenstrual syndrome (PMS).

Psychosocial stress may threaten sleep more than hormonal changes. Many young women reduce sleep to cope with work and their roles as mothers and wives. They ignore fatigue and other effects of inadequate sleep. A significant portion of employed women report sleep problems. Sleep problems are more common in women older than 40 years. Getting enough sleep improves job performance, concentration, social interaction, and general sense of well-being. Pregnancy may also disturb sleep. During the first trimester, women need more sleep and feel sleepier during the day. During the second trimester, sleep improves. During the third trimester, women sleep less and are more awake. The most common reasons for sleep disturbances are frequent urination, heartburn, general discomfort, fetal movements, low back pain, leg cramps, and nightmares. Swelling in nasal passages may cause snoring and sleep apnea during pregnancy. After childbirth, the irregular sleep pattern of the newborn can also significantly impact the mother's sleep.

As women age, physical and hormonal changes make sleep lighter and less sound. Sleep disturbances become more common during menopause. Women wake up more often at night and are more tired during the day. Hot flashes and night sweats linked to lower levels of estrogen may contribute to these problems. During the menopausal years, snoring becomes more frequent. After menopause, women get less deep sleep and are more likely to awaken at night than during menopause. There is also an increase on obstructive sleep apnea in post-menopausal women.

Pain, grief, worry, certain medical conditions, medications, and breathing disorders may disturb sleep in menopausal and postmenopausal women.

The most common sleep problem in women is insomnia. This includes trouble falling asleep, staying asleep, or early awakening, and inability to resume sleep. Other common sleep disorders are sleep-disordered breathing, restless legs syndrome, periodic limb movement disorder, and narcolepsy.

• Sleep-disordered breathing occurs with loud snoring, interrupted breathing during sleep, disrupted sleep, and daytime sleepiness. Sleep apnea increases in women older than 50 years.

• Restless legs syndrome (RLS) and periodic limb movement disorder (PLMD) can disturb sleep profoundly. The causes of these conditions are unknown, but it is often associated with low iron stores in the body. RLS occurs before sleep starts is more pronounced in the evening with an urge to move the legs. RLS causes calf discomfort and restlessness in the legs that is relieved by movement. PLMD causes periodic leg movements that may awaken the person from sleep. RLS may cause insomnia. PLMD may cause excessive sleepiness. Both conditions are more common in older people.

• Narcolepsy is an uncommon form of hypersomnia characterized by excessive daytime sleepiness. The major features of narcolepsy are sleep attacks and cataplexy. Sleep attacks are an irresistible urge to sleep. Cataplexy is a sudden loss of muscle tone typically preceded by emotional states. Other narcolepsy symptoms are sleep paralysis and hypnagogic hallucinations. Patients with narcolepsy often have disrupted sleep.

What Causes Sleep Disorders in Women?

• The changing hormonal levels during the menstrual cycle can disturb sleep and cause daytime sleepiness. Hormonal effects can be direct, by changing sleep patterns, or indirect, by affecting mood and emotional state. As many as 80% of women report premenstrual symptoms.

- Decreasing menopausal estrogen levels may cause hot flashes that disturb sleep. About two-thirds of menopausal women have sleep problems. Lower menopausal estrogen levels are linked with increased snoring risk and sleep-disordered breathing.

- In today's society, many women cope with the roles of wife, mother, caregiver for parents, and worker. With less time for themselves, they often reduce sleep. The sleep deprivation and stress are linked with long-term insomnia.

- Work and lifestyle can also contribute to primary sleep disorders. Women who work in rotating and night shifts are likely to experience sleep problems. Inactivity and lack of exercise can lead to trouble falling asleep. Women with erratic schedules or altered weekend sleep patterns are more likely to have trouble resetting their body clock to normal.

- Caffeine, nicotine, or other stimulating drugs near bedtime may prevent a woman from falling asleep. Alcohol may cause sleep fragmentation and nightmares.

- Depression and anxiety are more prevalent in women than in men and can contribute to sleep disorders. In some women, these are related to the menstrual cycle. Anxiety may impair falling asleep, and depression may cause early morning awakening.

- Sleep-disordered breathing is common in postmenopausal women. Multiple breathing cessations during sleep occur with sleep apnea. The resulting breathing difficulty disturbs sleep and may cause daytime fatigue. Sleep apnea is linked to high blood pressure and cardiovascular disease.

- Snoring often indicates partial airway obstruction. Snoring is linked with high blood pressure and increased risk for sleep apnea. Snoring increases during pregnancy, particularly during the last trimester. It is linked to pregnancy-related high blood pressure, preeclampsia, and low infant birth weight. Pregnant women do not have a higher risk of sleep-disordered breathing, and it is important for pregnant women who snore or are extremely tired to be evaluated. Untreated sleep apnea can be dangerous for both the mother and her unborn child.

• Sleep disorders are more common in older women.

• Being overweight or obese increases a woman's risk of having a sleep disorder.

What Are the Symptoms of Sleep Disorders in Women?

There are 3 common sleep disorder symptoms. Overlap is common.

• Difficulty falling asleep: This problem is more common in younger women. It is often linked to anxiety disorders and a stressful lifestyle.

• Difficulties maintaining sleep: Multiple awakenings during sleep are more common in older women. This symptom may indicate periodic limb movement disorder (PLMD). Arthritis, pain, medications, and the last trimester of pregnancy may cause multiple awakenings during sleep.

• Excessive daytime sleepiness: In older postmenopausal women, PLMD and sleep-disordered breathing may cause excessive daytime sleepiness. Sleep deprivation and narcolepsy are more likely to cause severe sleepiness in younger women.

What Exams and Tests Diagnose Sleep Disorders in Women?

If you are having sleeping problems, the first step is a detailed medical interview. You will be asked about your medical and psychological problems, physical symptoms, medications, family medical problems, menstrual and pregnancy history, work life, habits, and lifestyle. The next step is a physical examination.

Sleep Study

- Polysomnography: Overnight sleep studies or polysomnograms may be done in a sleep disorders center, at home, or in a hospital. Depending on the type of testing performed, the machine records EEG (sleep patterns) breathing patterns, ECG, eye movements, and changes in muscle tone.

- Multiple sleep latency test (MSLT): MSLT measures the level of daytime sleepiness. It is performed during the day following a supervised overnight polysomnogram.

- Sleep log: A sleep log is a diary of your sleep-wake cycles. You will be asked to keep a 2-week diary of sleep and daytime sleepiness. This diary can be helpful in diagnosing circadian rhythm disorders as well as irregular sleep patterns.

What Is the Treatment for Sleep Disorders in Women?

Medication may help in some women, but often behavior and lifestyle changes best relieve sleep problems.

Self-Care at Home for Sleep Disorders in Women

Guidelines For Better Sleep Hygiene

Sleep hygiene refers to habits and lifestyle that promote healthy sleep. Your health care provider will often recommend improved sleep hygiene.

• Try to wake up at the same time every day, regardless of the time you went to bed.

• Try to stay away from long daytime naps, but a brief regular daily nap may be helpful.

• Exercise daily but not in the hours before bedtime.

• Use the bed only for sleeping or sex.

• Do not read or watch television in bed.

• Do not use bedtime as worry time.

- Eat a balanced diet with regular mealtimes.

- Avoid heavy or spicy meals at bedtime.

- Avoid alcohol, caffeine, and nicotine before bedtime.

- Spend time right before bed relaxing and engaging is soothing activities.

- Develop a routine for getting ready for bed.

- Control the nighttime environment with comfortable temperature, noise, and light levels.

• Wear comfortable, loose-fitting clothes to bed.

• If unable to sleep within 30 minutes, get out of bed and perform a soothing activity, such as listening to soft music or reading. Avoid bright light exposure during these times.

• Get adequate exposure to bright light during the day.

Weight loss may help overweight, habitual, loud snorers. Alcohol and sedatives before bed may aggravate snoring. Also, avoid sleeping on your back. Taping a tennis ball to the back of your bedclothes may prevent you from sleeping on your back.

What Is the Medical Treatment for Sleep Disorders in Women?

Why doesn't your health care provider prescribe a sleeping pill for you? One reason is that sleeping pills may cause dependency and abuse. Also, sleeping pills may cause side effects and complications, such as confusion, dizziness, imbalance, falls, and a daytime "hangover." These medications are only a short-term solution. The dose for prescription sleeping pills was recently changed for women because of significant side effects.

Your health care provider may treat medical or psychological sleep disorders or refer you to a specialist. Your health care provider may also change or discontinue medications to improve sleep. The treatment for sleep-disordered breathing is continuous positive airway pressure (CPAP). A mask is worn over the nose or mouth while you sleep, and gentle steady air pressure from the mask keeps your airway open. CPAP often provides immediate relief. Patients feel more rested at night and are more alert during the day.

What Medications Treat Sleep Disorders in Women?

Health care providers use short-term and long-term drug treatment to treat sleep disorders. Sleep medications are a short-term drug treatment for insomnia. Other names for sleeping medications are hypnotics or sedatives. The goal is to reduce insomnia without sacrificing daytime alertness. Short-term treatment lasts 2-4 weeks. The health care provider treats the underlying cause of the sleep disorder during this period.

The most widely used sleep medications are the benzodiazepine and nonbenzodiazepine drugs. Tolerance develops quickly, and over time, a higher dose is required to get the same effect as the initial dose. The risk of becoming dependent on these medications is high. These medications may cause withdrawal symptoms. These are the reasons for using sleep medications on a short-term basis. Examples are the benzodiazepines lorazepam (Ativan), triazolam (Halcion), and temazepam (Restoril) and the nonbenzodiazepines zolpidem (Ambien) and zaleplon (Sonata).Ramelteon (Rozerem) is a prescription drug that stimulates melatonin receptors. A newer classification of medications for treating insomnia includes Suvorexant (Belsomra).

Melatonin is a hormone produced by the pineal gland during the dark hours of the day-night cycle (circadian rhythm). Melatonin levels in the body are low during daylight hours. The pineal gland (located in the brain) responds to darkness by increasing melatonin levels in the body. This process is thought to be integral to maintaining circadian rhythm. Ramelteon promotes the onset of sleep and helps normalize circadian rhythm disorders. Ramelteon is approved by the Food and Drug Administration (FDA) for insomnia characterized by difficulty falling asleep. Long-term treatment consists of treating medical and psychological conditions that underlie sleep disorders. In some cases, the sleep disorder is treated directly.

Hormone replacement therapy (HRT) improves sleep in menopausal women. HRT reduces hot flashes that disturb sleep. HRT may also improve sleep-related breathing disorders. HRT may be estrogen alone, or estrogen with progesterone. HRT is not for every woman, but it can markedly improve menopause symptoms. Long-term use of HRT involves risks. Make sure you understand the risks and benefits before you start HRT. Antidepressant drugs are sometimes used for women with chronic (long-term) insomnia. These drugs usually work, even in people who have no other depression. They also help some premenstrual sleep problems, postpartum depression, anxiety-related sleep disorders, and clinical depression. They alter brain chemicals called neurotransmitters, such as serotonin and norepinephrine. These drugs do not cause dependency. Examples are sertraline (Zoloft), fluoxetine (Sarafem or Prozac), and mirtazapine (Remeron). Stimulants are sometimes used to treat narcolepsy. These drugs promote wakefulness. An example is modafinil (Provigil). Dopamine agonists are drugs that promote release of the neurotransmitter dopamine in the brain. These drugs may improve restless legs syndrome. An example is pramipexole (Mirapex).

Is There Surgery For Sleep Disorders In Women?

Uvulopalatopharyngoplasty (UPPP) is one operation that eliminates loud snoring and obstruction in some cases. The surgeon repositions tissues to enlarge and stabilize the throat opening and prevent airflow obstruction. Other procedures may be considered as well if an examination reveals an appropriate indication.

What Is the Followup for Sleep Disorders in Women?

Your health care provider will ask you to return in a few weeks to see if treatment is effective. Regular visits are necessary if you take medication or receive sleep apnea treatment.

How Do You Prevent Sleep Disorders in Women?

Good sleep habits will improve insomnia and frequent sleep awakenings. Managing stress and maintaining a healthy weight help women sleep better and prevent more serious sleep problems.

What Is the Prognosis for Sleep Disorders in Women?

Persistent insomnia may cause daytime fatigue, decreased daytime function, memory and concentration problems, depression, and injuries and accidents. Women with persistent insomnia tend to have more psychological and medical problems. The outlook for persistent insomnia is good if the underlying problem is treated. Untreated or undertreated sleep apnea may cause heart rhythm problems, high blood pressure, and congestive heart failure. Daytime fatigue from sleep apnea increases the risk of accidents and injuries. Effectively treated sleep apnea has an excellent prognosis. CPAP treatment improves alertness, nocturnal awakenings, and sense of well-being.

Cure Your Sleep Disorder With Natural Treatments

The treatments for sleep disorders today can be generally grouped into three categories: behavioral or psychotherapeutic treatments, sleep medications or drugs and treatments that don't fit into the other two categories. The excessive sleep disorder narcolepsy will cause most patients to have unexpected periods of sleep throughout the day for as little as a few minutes to as long as half an hour at times. There are generally three types of sleep disorders: lack of enough sleep, sleep disturbance, and too much or excessive sleep. The person suffering from a sleep disorder may have difficulty getting to sleep at night or staying asleep as well as having difficulty staying awake through the day; they may also experience different types of behaviors that prevent them from staying asleep during their normal sleeping hours. One type of sleep disorder, lack of sleep, is also commonly known as insomnia and is what people usually have rather than a more complex sleeping disorder. Sleep apnea can be life threatening; this problem is usually accompanied by heavy and loud snoring and causes the person to wake up sometimes hundred of times during the night without remembering ever being awake. In the excessive sleep disorder type the most well-known is called narcolepsy. Finding that you need coffee, colas or other caffeine drinks throughout the day to stay alert or awake can also be a hint that sleep disorder treatments need to be investigated. There are number of sleep disorders that appear in different people and even those with similar sleep disorders often display different symptoms. Many people say they survive nicely on four or five hours of sleep; others say they need nine or even ten hours. The sleep disorder narcolepsy can have complications such as cataplexy and hypnagogic hallucinations; cataplexy is the weakness or complete paralysis of the muscles, and hypnagogic hallucinations are vivid dreams that happen during the stage of sleep between being awake and being asleep. Delayed Sleep Phase Syndrome is a sleep disorder of circadian rhythm, characterized by the inability to wake up and fall asleep at the desired times, but not by the inability to stay asleep. Periodic Limb Movement Disorder (PLMD) is the involuntary movement of arms and/or legs during sleep. Narcolepsy is the sleep disorder of falling asleep spontaneously and unwillingly. Don't get into the habit of drinking a glass of wine, hard liquor, or any other alcoholic beverage at bedtime; alcohol is a central nervous system depressant and it will interfere with your REM (rapid eye movement) sleep and cause other problems you might not be aware of. Some health experts suggest that contracting then relaxing all your muscles starting with your toes and proceeding upwards as you lie in bed can help you relax. In bed do try to focus on anything pleasant, long enough to distract you from any worries that are keeping you awake. Some people say that sleeping with your head facing north helps you fall asleep because your body is better aligned with the earth. Concentrating on some of the insomnia tips you've heard in the past may put your mind at rest long enough to allow you to go to sleep. Your pillow may make you feel as though you're lying uphill or downhill and if it is too hard may press into your head uncomfortably, reducing the chance of your falling asleep. In some sleep tests they used a flashlight to shine light on the back of the knee and tested the reaction of the brain on the sleeping centers and the light was detected; your body knows when there is a light shining on the back side of your body. Make sure that you don't have any light on in the bedroom, including the red light on digital clocks, night lights or any other light, even a small flicker; any light at all can stop the production of melatonin which is produced when it starts getting dark enough in your bedroom but may shut down if even the smallest light is glowing. You need to produce melatonin for a good nights sleep. If you lie in bed struggling with the day's stresses and worries, try some of the insomnia tips you've heard over the years such as counting sheep or visualizing a blank screen. Some doctors may offer sleeping medications as a short-term solution along with some insomnia tips, but will seek to find the underlying cause of the sleeplessness and treat the cause instead of the symptom. Among the many insomnia tips provided by doctors and other health professionals, the most important tip is the ability to get physically relaxed enough to fall asleep. Finding the solution to your sleeping problems or sleep disorder will be worth the investment in time. Your doctor or sleep specialist may be able to recommend support groups to you. Consider going to a sleep disorder center because they provide the newest research for the many issues that involve any sleep disorder.

8 Home Remedies for Sleeping Disorder

Many people experience short-term insomnia. This common sleep disorder can make it difficult to fall asleep and stay asleep until it's time to wake up.

Although the amount of sleep needed varies from person to person, most adults need at least seven hours of sleep a night. If your sleeping patterns are affecting your quality of life, home remedies may be able to help.

Keep reading to learn how you can take charge of your sleeping patterns through meditation, exercise, and other home remedies.

Mindfulness Meditation

Mindfulness meditation consists of slow, steady breathing while sitting quietly. You observe your breath, body, thoughts, feelings, and sensations as they rise and pass.

Mindfulness meditation has numerous health benefits that go hand-in-hand with a healthy lifestyle promoting good sleep. It's said to reduce stress, improve concentration, and boost immunity.

Researchers in a 2011 studyTrusted Source found that meditation significantly improved insomnia and overall sleep patterns. Participants attended a weekly meditation class, a daylong retreat, and practiced at home over the course of a few months.

You can meditate as often as you like. If you don't have time for a longer session, aim to do 15 minutes in the morning or evening. Consider joining a meditation group once a week to stay motivated. You may also choose to do an online guided meditation.

Meditation is safe to practice, but it has the potential to bring up strong emotions. If you feel it is causing you further angst or turmoil, discontinue the practice.

Mantra Repetition

Repeating a mantra or positive affirmation repeatedly can help focus and calm your mind. Mantras are said to produce feelings of relaxation by quieting the mind.

Researchers in a 2015 study taught women who are homeless to repeat a mantra silently throughout the day and before sleeping. Participants who continued to use the mantra over the course of a week experienced reduced levels of insomnia.

You may choose a mantra in Sanskrit, English, or another language. Search online for ideas or create one that feels right for you. Choose a mantra that you find pleasant and calming. It should be a simple, positive statement in the present tense. A good mantra will allow you to continually focus on the repetition of sound, which will enable you to relax and go to sleep.

Chant the mantra mentally or aloud, keeping your focus on the words. Gently bring your mind back to the mantra each time it wanders. You may also play music with chanting. Feel free to recite your mantra as often as you like. You might choose another mantra to use in the daytime.

If you feel the chanting is causing any ill effects or agitation, stop the practice.

Yoga

Yoga has been found as a trusted Source to have a positive effect on sleep quality. Yoga may also alleviate stress, improve physical functioning, and boost mental focus.

Choose a style that focuses more on moving meditation or breath work as opposed to difficult physical movements. Slow, controlled movements allow you to stay present and focused. Yin and restorative yoga are great options.

Strive to do a few longer sessions each week, and at least 20 minutes of daily self-practice. Performing the postures before bed can help you to relax and unwind.

If a pose doesn't feel right for you, don't force it. Forcing it may result in injury. It's important to do what feels good for you and your body, and that varies from person to person.

Exercise

Exercise boosts overall health. It can enhance your mood, give you more energy, aid in weight loss, and promote better sleep.

Participants in a 2015 study, exercised for at least 150 minutes per week for six months. During this time, researchers found that the participants experienced significantly fewer symptoms of insomnia. They also showed reduced symptoms of depression and anxiety.

To receive these benefits, you should engage in moderate exercise for at least 20 minutes per day. You may add in some strength training or vigorous aerobic exercise a few times per week. Find the time of day that best suits your needs and that has the most positive effect on your sleep.

Take into consideration the condition of your body and exercise accordingly. Physical injury is possible, but can usually be avoided if you practice with care.

Massage

Researchers in a 2015 found massage therapy to benefit people with insomnia by improving sleep quality and daytime dysfunction. It may also reduce feelings of pain, anxiety, and depression.

If professional massage isn't an option, you can do self-massage. You may also find it beneficial to have a partner or friend give you a massage. Allow your mind to focus on the feelings and sensations of touch as your mind wanders. Research online for tips and techniques.

While massage is generally safe, check with your doctor if you have any specific health concerns that may impede the benefits. If your skin is sensitive to creams or oils, be sure to do a skin patch test before use.

Magnesium

Magnesium is a naturally occurring mineral. It can help muscles relax and relieve stress. This is thought to encourage healthy sleep patterns.

Participants in a 2012 took 500 milligrams (mg) of magnesium daily for 2 months. During this time, researchers found that participants experienced fewer symptoms of insomnia and improved sleep patterns.

Men may take up to 400 mg daily, and women can take up to 300 mg daily. You may choose to divide your doses between the morning and evening or take your dose before bed.

You may also add 1 cup of magnesium flakes to your evening bath, allowing the magnesium to be absorbed through your skin.

Side effects include stomach and intestinal issues. You may wish to start with a lower dose and gradually increase to see how your body reacts. Taking it with food may reduce any abdominal discomfort. Check with your doctor if you take any medications to determine potential interactions.

You shouldn't take magnesium supplements constantly. Take a break for a few days every two weeks. Don't take more than the recommended dose found on the product.

Lavender oil

Lavender is used to improve mood, reduce pain, and promote sleep. Taking it orally is thought to be more effective.

Results of a 2014 study showed that lavender oil capsules were beneficial in improving sleep patterns in people with depression when taken with an antidepressant. People also showed lowered levels of anxiety, which would seemingly allow for better sleep.

Take 20 to 80 mg of lavender orally each day, or use as directed. You may wish to add lavender essential oil to a diffuser or spray it onto your pillow. Lavender tea is also an option.

Lavender is usually safe to use. Taking lavender orally may cause headache, constipation, or nausea.

Check out: What lavender can do for you »

Remedy #8: Melatonin

Melatonin can help you to fall asleep more quickly and enhance the quality of your sleep.

Researchers in a 2016 studyTrusted Source found melatonin to significantly improve sleep patterns in people with cancer and insomnia. Sleep quality was improved even more between seven and 14 days.

Take 1 to 5 mg 30 minutes to two hours before going to sleep. You should use the lowest effective dose possible, as higher doses may cause side effects.

It may cause:

depression

dizziness

headaches

irritability

stomach cramps

wakefulness in the night

Melatonin is generally safe to use for short periods of time.

What else can I do to help sleep through the night?

Certain lifestyle changes may also help reduce your symptoms of insomnia. You may wish to give these a shot before seeking out supplemental or medicinal options.

Tips and tricks

Avoid chemicals that disrupt sleep, such as nicotine, caffeine, and alcohol.

Eat lighter meals at night and at least two hours before bed.

Stay active, but exercise earlier in the day.

Take a hot shower or bath at the end
of your day.

Avoid screens one to two hours before
bed.

Keep your bedroom dark and cool, and
try to use it only for sleeping.

Get into bed only if you're tired.

Get out of bed if you don't fall asleep
within 20 minutes.

When to see a doctor

If your symptoms persist for more
than a few weeks or worsen, consult

your doctor. Persistent insomnia may be the result of an underlying health concern.

This includes:

heartburn

diabetes

asthma

arthritis

chronic pain

thyroid disease

cardiovascular disease

musculoskeletal disorders

kidney disease

neurological disorders

respiratory problems

hormonal changes associated with menopause

Prescription and over-the-counter medications may also interfere with sleep quality.

If left untreated, insomnia can increase your risk for:

anxiety

depression

heart failure

high blood pressure

substance abuse

Your doctor can help you to get to the root cause and decide how best to treat the issue.

How is insomnia traditionally treated?

If lifestyle changes aren't working, your doctor may suggest behavioral therapy.

Behavioral therapy

Behavioral therapy can help you to develop habits that improve the quality of your sleep. Your therapist will work with you over the course of a few months to figure out which thoughts and behaviors are contributing negatively to your sleep patterns.

A cognitive behavioral treatment plan may include:

sleep restriction

relaxation therapy

sleep hygiene education

sleep scheduling

stimulus control

This usually has better long-term outcomes than medicine alone.

Medication

Sleeping medication should only be used occasionally and for no more than 10 consecutive days.

Over-the-counter options include diphenhydramine, such as in Benadryl, and doxylamine succinate, such as in Unisom SleepTabs.

Your doctor may prescribe sleeping pills to be used while you're adjusting to behavior and lifestyle changes.

Common prescription sleep medicines include:

doxepin (Silenor)

eszopiclone (Lunesta)

zolpidem (Ambien)

Learn more: Lunesta vs. Ambien, two short-term treatments for insomnia »

Outlook

In many cases, making positive changes to your lifestyle can relieve insomnia. Infrequent insomnia typically lasts for a few days or weeks. In more severe cases, it can last three months or longer. If your symptoms persist for more than a few weeks, consult your doctor.

You may find it beneficial to have plan for what to do when you can't sleep. You may decide to focus on relaxing in bed without sleeping, move to another room to do something relaxing, or get up and do something more active and productive. Find what works for you.

Keeping a sleep journal may help you identify any factors contributing to your insomnia. Be sure to record your nighttime routine, anything you had to eat or drink, and any medications you

may be taking.